ESSENTIAL 101 TIPS

Healthy

PREGNANCY

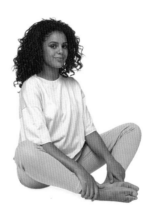

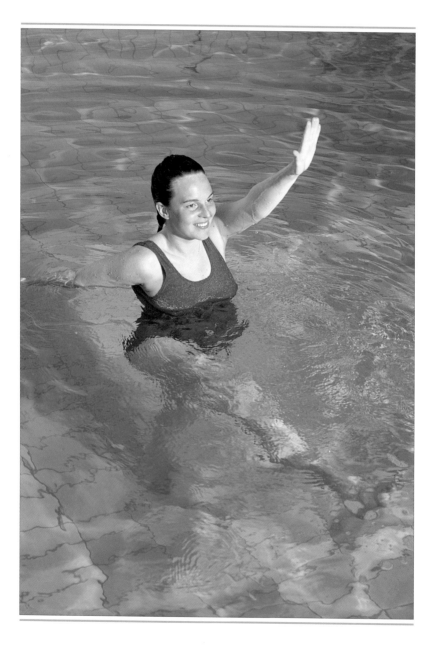

ESSENTIAL 101 TIPS

Healthy
PREGNANCY

Elizabeth Fenwick

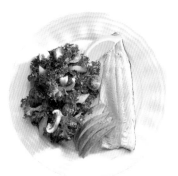

DK PUBLISHING, INC.

www.dk.com

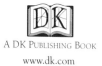

A DK PUBLISHING BOOK

www.dk.com

Editor Alexa Stace
Art Editor Ann Burnham
DTP Designer Mark Bracey
Series Editor Charlotte Davies
Series Art Editor Clive Hayball
Production Controller Lauren Britton

First American Edition, 1996
6 8 10 9 7

Published in the United States by DK Publishing, Inc.,
95 Madison Avenue, New York, New York 10016

ISBN 0-7894-1078-8

Text film output by The Right Type, Great Britain
Reproduced by Colourscan, Singapore
Printed by Wing King Tong, Hong Kong

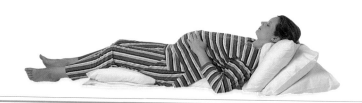

ESSENTIAL TIPS

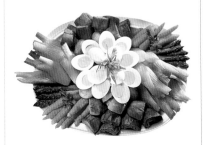

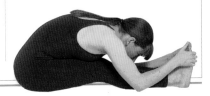

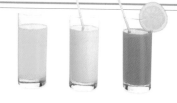
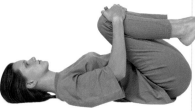
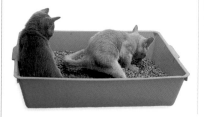

PREPARING FOR LABOR

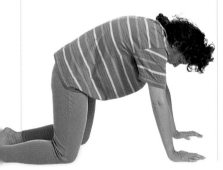

COMMON COMPLAINTS

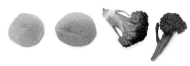

AFTER THE BIRTH

ACKNOWLEDGMENTS 72

THINKING ABOUT PREGNANCY

1 CHECKLIST FOR A HEALTHY PREGNANCY

If possible, plan for pregnancy at least three months before you conceive. It is in the first few weeks, when you may not even know you are pregnant, that the baby's development can be most easily affected. Staying healthy and eating well will make sure that you nourish and protect the baby in the womb. Answer the questions below on potential risks, and consult your doctor before you start trying to conceive.

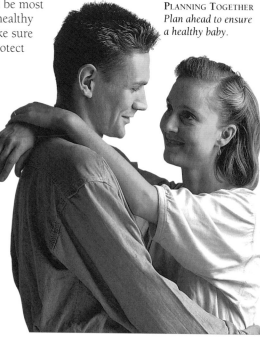

PLANNING TOGETHER
Plan ahead to ensure a healthy baby.

CHECKLIST
- *Have you had German measles?* (see p.29)
- *Do you or your partner have a family history of inherited disease such as hemophilia? If so, consult your doctor.*
- *Do you have a medical condition such as diabetes or epilepsy? If so, consult your doctor.*
- *Does your work bring you into contact with any risks?* (see p.11)
- *Do you smoke or drink?* (see p.10)
- *Are you on the pill?* (see right)

MILK ▷
*A balanced
diet should
include
calcium – milk
is a good source.*

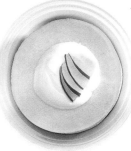

2 A HEALTHY DIET

A baby's health depends to a great extent on the health of both parents at the time of conception. You and your partner will increase your chances of conceiving, and of giving birth to a healthy baby, if you eat a healthy, varied diet. It should be low in fats and should include a good selection of fresh vegetables and raw fruit.

△ FRESH FRUIT
*Fresh melon with yogurt
and nectarines makes a
delicious dessert to round
out a balanced meal.*

NUTRITIOUS MEAL ▷
*Make sure you eat enough
protein and fresh vegetables
every day. This dish of
poached salmon and
salad is ideal.*

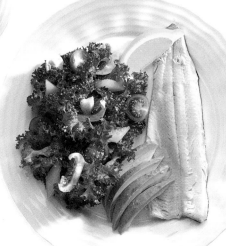

3 GIVING UP THE PILL

If you are on the pill, it is best to stop taking it well before you want to conceive, to allow your body time to return to its normal cycle. Ideally, you should wait until you have had three normal menstrual periods before trying to become pregnant (you can use a condom or diaphragm during this time). If you conceive before the regular rhythm of your periods has been established again, it makes it more difficult to predict the delivery date of your baby.

9

4 SMOKING

Smoking is one of the most damaging factors to the health of your unborn baby. If you are a smoker, you should give up before you try to conceive. Mothers who smoke are more likely to have premature and underweight babies. Smoking also increases the chances of miscarriage, stillbirth, or malformity. Even after birth, the baby of a smoker has a higher risk of SIDS (Sudden Infant Death Syndrome).

The more you smoke, the greater the risk to the baby

Smoking deprives the baby of oxygen, and increases the risk of miscarriage, stillbirth, and fetal abnormalities

The babies of smokers are more likely to be premature, and to have a low birthweight. A parent who smokes increases the risk of SIDS.

PASSIVE SMOKING
Breathing in the smoke from other people's cigarettes can also damage the health of your baby, so encourage your partner to give up smoking too. Young children whose parents smoke are more likely to develop bronchitis and asthma, and they can suffer impaired growth.

Cramping pains in the legs when walking are a warning sign of impaired circulation, caused by smoking

5 DRINKING

Drinking heavily can affect the fertility of both men and women, and can also seriously affect the development of the baby in the womb. No one knows what the safe level of drinking is in this case, so give up alcohol completely while you are trying to conceive, or at least cut down your alcohol intake to the recommended maximum of two units per day. Avoid hard liquor altogether.

6 DANGEROUS SUBSTANCES

If you or your partner has a job that involves working with chemicals, lead, anesthetics, or X-rays, this may affect your chances of conceiving or involve a risk to the unborn baby, so talk to your doctor. Also avoid inhaling fumes from cleaning fluids, oven cleaners, paint, lacquers, gasoline, and glue.

7 VDTS

It used to be thought that computers, VDTs, and copying machines gave off harmful rays, but there is no evidence that they present any risk to pregnant women or their babies. If using a computer, you should sit comfortably in front of a screen, in a chair with enough support, to avoid back and shoulder strain.

8 TAKING DRUGS & MEDICINES

Some drugs and medicines may affect your chances of becoming pregnant, or harm the baby in the womb. If you regularly take any medication, for disorders such as epilepsy or diabetes, for example, talk with your doctor before you try to conceive. With many drugs, the long-term effects on the fetus are unknown. Drugs that have been proved to be hazardous should be avoided completely, and all others should be viewed with suspicion.

Drugs to avoid

Drug	Use	Fetal effect
Accutane	Acne	Causes birth defects
Amphetamines	Stimulant	Heart defects
Antihistamines	Allergies	Possible malformations
Antinausea	Sickness	Possible malformations
Aspirin	Painkiller	Prevents blood clotting
Codeine	Painkiller	Addictive
Diuretics	Weight loss	Blood disorders
Phenytoin	Epilepsy	Malformations
Steroids	Various	Hormonal
Streptomycin	Infections	Deafness
Sulfonamides	Infections	Birth jaundice
Tetracycline	Infections	Discoloration of teeth
Valium	Anxiety	Respiratory problems

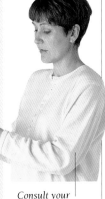

Consult your doctor before taking any drug

9 WEIGHT & EXERCISE

Ideally, your weight should be normal for your height for at least six months before conceiving, so if you are seriously over- or underweight, see your doctor for advice on attaining the right weight. Unless you have a serious weight problem, never diet in pregnancy, as you may deprive your body of vital nutrients. To keep yourself in shape while you are trying to conceive, try to get some form of exercise, such as walking or swimming, for at least 20 minutes each day.

6% increase in weight of breasts

29% baby

6% placenta

8% amniotic fluid

8% increase in weight of uterus

25% extra fat and fluid retention

16% increase in blood volume

WEIGHT GAIN IN PREGNANCY
How much you gain will depend on how much you weigh beforehand. A woman of average build will probably gain 20–30 lb (10–13.5 kg). The pregnancy accounts for about 16–18 lb (8–9 kg) of total weight gained, so any excess will remain after delivery. Try hard to walk or swim every day to stay in shape, but don't diet.

GAINING TOO MUCH WEIGHT
Even if you put on too much weight, do not go on a diet. Cut down on sugary or fatty foods. Snack on fruit and healthy foods rather than cake, cookies, or cheese, which are high in calories. A sudden excessive weight gain after the 30th week may be a sign of preeclampsia.

ESSENTIAL NUTRIENTS

10 EATING FOR A HEALTHY BABY

A baby has only one source of food –
you. During pregnancy it is essential that
you have as varied and balanced a diet as
possible. This does not mean planning a
special diet or eating for two. All you
have to do is eat a variety of fresh,
unprocessed foods (a selection is given
on pages 14–23), to ensure you get all the
nutrients you need. Once you are
pregnant, consider everything that you
eat or drink that might harm the
baby (*see pp.36–37*). Increase
your intake of raw vegetables
and fresh fruit, and reduce
that of sugary, salty, and
processed foods.

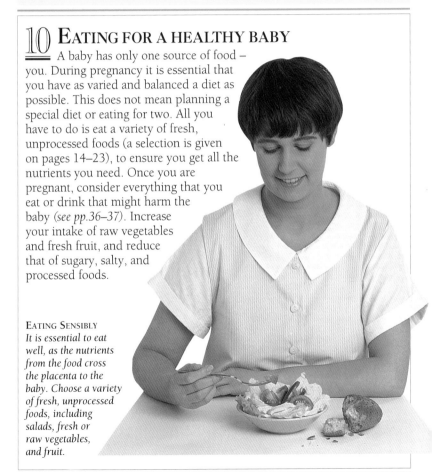

EATING SENSIBLY
*It is essential to eat
well, as the nutrients
from the food cross
the placenta to the
baby. Choose a variety
of fresh, unprocessed
foods, including
salads, fresh or
raw vegetables,
and fruit.*

11 CALCIUM

In order to ensure the healthy development of your baby's bones and teeth, which start to form from about week eight, you will need about twice as much calcium as normal. Good sources include cheese, milk, yogurt, and leafy green vegetables. However, dairy products are also high in fat, so if you are gaining too much weight choose lowfat varieties, such as skim or lowfat milk, yogurt, and cottage cheese rather than whole-milk cheeses.

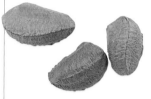

SKIM MILK ▷
Dairy products are high in fat, so skim or lowfat milk is a better option if you are gaining a lot of weight.

BRAZIL NUTS △
Nuts are a good source of calcium but high in fat.

SARDINES △
Just 6oz (180g) of sardines will give you the extra calcium you need in a day.

◁ LOWFAT CHEESE
Eat lowfat or cottage cheese since cheese is high in fat and calories.

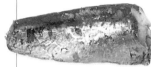

FROMAGE FRAIS △
Fromage frais and farmer cheese are good choices as they are lowfat.

◁ WHITE BREAD
If you do not eat fish or dairy foods, try enriched white bread as a source of calcium.

12 PROTEIN

As your nutritional needs increase during your pregnancy, try to eat a variety of foods rich in protein. Poultry, nuts, fish, meat, rice, beans, and dairy products all supply protein. Try to limit your intake of red meat as it is also high in fat; choose lean cuts whenever possible (venison is a very lean red meat). Poultry is low in fat, particularly if you remove the skin before cooking.

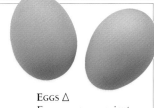

EGGS △
Eggs are a convenient form of protein.

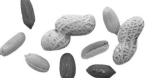

PEANUTS △
Nuts are a valuable source of protein.

HARD CHEESE ▷
Hard cheeses such as cheddar are high in protein as well as calcium, but limit your intake because of the high fat content.

PEANUT BUTTER △
A peanut butter sandwich makes a high-protein snack.

LENTILS △
Dried lentils, beans, including soy beans and soy milk, and peas are high in protein.

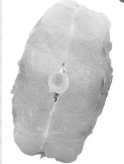

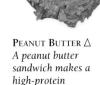

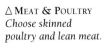

FISH △
Fish is a good source of protein; it is low in fat and easy to digest.

△ **MEAT & POULTRY**
Choose skinned poultry and lean meat.

13 VITAMIN C

Vitamin C will help to build a strong placenta, assist your body in resisting infection, and aid the absorption of iron. It is found in fresh fruit and vegetables, and supplies are needed daily, since it cannot be stored in the body. Prolonged storage and cooking of produce destroys its vitamin C.

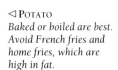

RED & GREEN PEPPERS ▷
Eat these fresh vegetables raw whenever possible for maximum benefit.

◁ POTATO
Baked or boiled are best. Avoid French fries and home fries, which are high in fat.

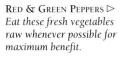

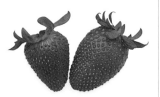

△ SAVOY CABBAGE & BRUSSELS SPROUTS
Steam green vegetables, or eat them raw if possible.

CAULIFLOWER △
Steam cauliflower to avoid destroying the vitamin content.

ORANGE △
Drink freshly squeezed orange juice for maximum vitamins.

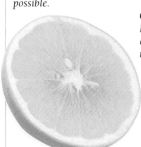

◁ GRAPEFRUIT
Grapefruit makes a healthy addition to your breakfast menu.

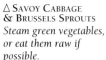

△ STRAWBERRIES
Serve them fresh with breakfast cereal.

14 FIBER

This should form a large part of your daily diet, since constipation *(see p.60)* is common in pregnancy. Fruit and vegetables are ideal sources of fiber that you can eat a lot of every day. Bread, pasta, and rice, especially brown rice, are also valuable sources, and dried fruit and nuts. Avoid too much bran as it can hinder the absorption of other nutrients.

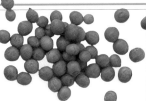

GARDEN PEAS △
All vegetables are high in fiber. Eat fresh or frozen peas, not processed.

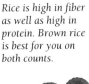

BROWN RICE ▷
Rice is high in fiber as well as high in protein. Brown rice is best for you on both counts.

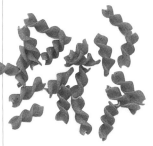

△ **WHOLE-WHEAT PASTA**
Pasta is a good source of carbohydrates and fibre. Eat whole-wheat pasta if possible.

◁ **RASPBERRIES**
Fresh fruit is high in fiber as well as vitamin C. Eat as much as you like, but avoid canned fruit in syrup.

WHOLE-GRAIN BREAD ▷
Make sandwiches from whole-grain bread as it is high in protein as well as fiber.

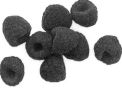

◁ **LEEKS**
Ideal for fiber as well as vitamin C and iron. Steam lightly.

15 IRON

The baby needs to build up stores of iron for early infancy, and the extra blood your body produces needs iron to carry oxygen. Iron from red meat is absorbed more easily than that from foods such as beans and dried fruit, so if you do not eat meat, combine iron-rich foods with those rich in vitamin C to aid absorption.

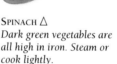

SPINACH △
Dark green vegetables are all high in iron. Steam or cook lightly.

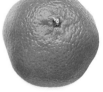

DRIED APRICOTS △
Dried fruits, particularly apricots and prunes, have a high iron content.

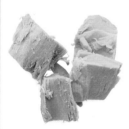

△ **TUNA**
All fish are high in iron and also have the advantage of being low in fat.

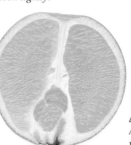

△ **ORANGES**
Always take vitamin C with iron-rich foods.

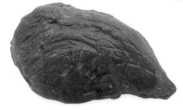

△ **LEAN RED MEAT**
Red meat is one of the best and most easily absorbed sources of iron. Try to choose lean cuts and avoid liver (see right).

16 LIVER WARNING

Liver is very high in vitamin A, which can be toxic to the fetus in large quantities. To be on the safe side, avoid liver and liver products, such as pâté and liver sausage, as well as vitamin A supplements.

17 FOLIC ACID

This is necessary for the development of the baby's central nervous system, especially in the first few weeks. All women in the childbearing years should take daily vitamins that include folic acid. The body cannot store this nutrient, so it is essential to have a daily supply. Fresh dark green vegetables, fruit, nuts, and seeds are all good sources. Folic acid is largely destroyed by cooking, so serve salads, and stir-fry or steam vegetables lightly.

◁ **PEANUTS**
All nuts are rich in folic acid, but avoid salted ones if possible.

HAZELNUTS ▷
Hazelnuts make a tasty snack.

◁ **BRUSSELS SPROUTS**
These are high in folic acid. Steam or shred in salads.

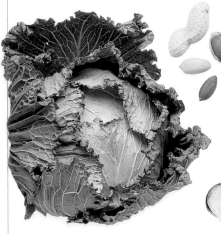

△ **LEAFY GREEN VEGETABLES**
Cooking destroys the nutrients, so steam or eat raw.

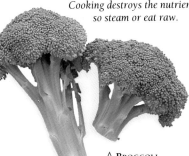

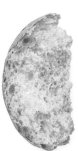

△ **BROCCOLI**
Steam lightly for maximum benefit.

△ **WHOLE-GRAIN BREAD**
Whole-grain breads are high in folic acid. Eat daily.

18 VITAMIN SUPPLEMENTS

Even if you eat a well-balanced diet, with plenty of fresh fruit and vegetables, you should take prenatal vitamins to make sure that you are getting all the minerals and vitamins you need. Iron supplements may be given if blood tests show that you are anemic.

19 CRAVINGS

It is common in pregnancy to find that you suddenly develop a great liking for certain foods, such as green olives or bananas, while others will repel you completely. This may be because rising hormone levels affect your saliva, making certain foods taste different from normal. If you do develop a craving for some particular food, go ahead and indulge yourself within reason, provided it is not too high in calories and low in nutrition, and does not cause indigestion.

◁ APPETITE IN PREGNANCY
You may experience unusual food cravings or dislike favorite foods.

20 FLUID

Your blood volume expands by nearly half during pregnancy, so it is important to keep up your fluid intake. Water is best; drink as much of it as you like. Fruit juices are good, but avoid ones with added sugar or artificial sweeteners.

DRINK MORE WATER

21 SALT

Most people consume too much salt in their diet. During pregnancy, it is particularly important to reduce your intake, since too much salt is related to problems such as swollen ankles and hands, and high blood pressure, which can be very dangerous.

REDUCE YOUR SALT INTAKE

22 VEGETARIAN DIETS

If you eat a variety of protein-rich foods and fresh fruit and vegetables every day, you should provide the baby with almost everything it needs. You may lack iron; the body has difficulty absorbing iron from plant sources. Prenatal vitamins ensure complete nutrition. To maximize absorption, combine iron-rich foods (*see p.18*) with foods rich in vitamin C (*see p.16*). If you are a vegan, you should also take calcium, and vitamins D and B12.

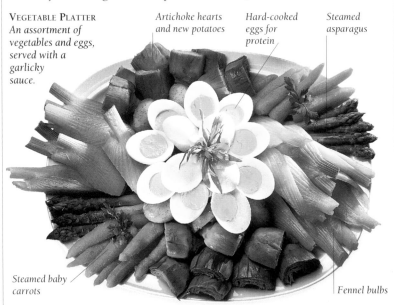

VEGETABLE PLATTER
An assortment of vegetables and eggs, served with a garlicky sauce.

Artichoke hearts and new potatoes

Hard-cooked eggs for protein

Steamed asparagus

Steamed baby carrots

Fennel bulbs

23 PROCESSED FOOD

Try to avoid convenience foods that have been highly processed, such as canned foods and packaged mixes. These often have added sugar and salt, as well as a high fat content. They also contain chemicals in the form of artificial flavorings, colorings, and preservatives. Additives in foods can be easily identified on the labels; avoid foods with artificial ingredients listed.

24 HEALTHY MEALS & SNACKS

Previous tips in this chapter have listed the various nutrients that are essential to the normal development of a healthy baby. Below we give some suggestions on how to combine these nutrients into healthy meals and snacks that you can serve to the whole family. None of them are difficult to prepare. You may not always have the time or inclination to cook elaborate meals such as stews or roasts, but it is still possible to eat well. Rice, pasta, legumes, fish, cheese, and egg dishes are all valuable, together with fresh vegetables and salads, whole-grain bread, and fresh fruit.

THREE-PEPPER PIZZA WITH CHEESE ▽
An ideal supper dish, the homemade pizza base is topped with sliced peppers, onions, parsley and other herbs sautéed in oil. Mozzarella cheese is then scattered on top and the pizza is baked for 20–25 minutes.

SANDWICH △
A chicken salad sandwich on whole-grain bread is an ideal choice for lunch or a quick snack.

PASTA ▽
An important source of carbohydrates and fiber.

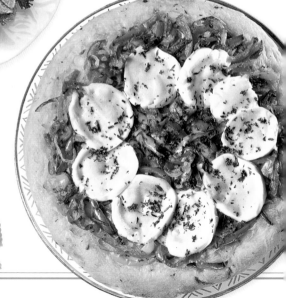

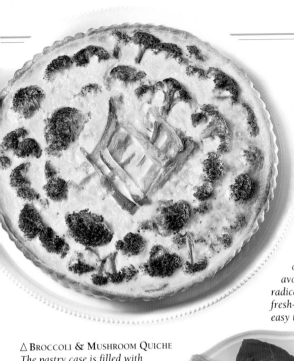

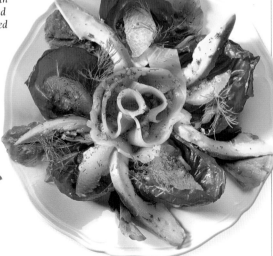

FRUIT △
Try to eat some
fresh fruit every
day.

▽ AVOCADO SALAD
This main course salad
of smoked salmon,
avocado, grapefruit, and
radicchio with dill dressing is
fresh-tasting, and quick and
easy to prepare.

△ BROCCOLI & MUSHROOM QUICHE
The pastry case is filled with
lightly steamed broccoli and
sautéed mushrooms, encased
in a tasty cheese custard.

WHOLE-GRAIN BREAD ▽
Two slices of whole-
grain bread provide
4 g of fiber.

PROTECTING YOU & YOUR BABY

25 WORKING WHEN PREGNANT

Many women continue working well into their pregnancy, and there is no reason not to, unless the work environment is a risk to your health or the baby (see p.11). If you are in a smoking environment, transfer to a smoke-free zone if possible. Make sure you get plenty of rest at home and at lunchtime to combat increasing fatigue and the stress of commuting to work. Relax your standards at home; your health is more important than an immaculate house.

COPING AT WORK
- *Sit down as much as possible, and put your feet up if you can.*
- *Do a few neck and shoulder relaxation exercises.*
- *Squat or kneel rather than bend down (see p.40).*
- *Keep a supply of nutritious snacks handy (see right).*
- *Don't push yourself too hard: take a rest when you get home, and let household chores slide.*
- *Ask your partner for help with cooking and cleaning.*

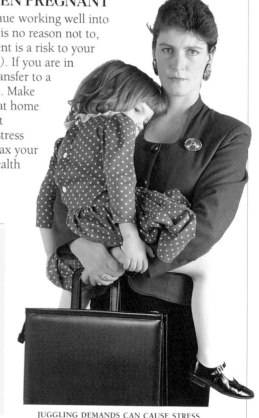

JUGGLING DEMANDS CAN CAUSE STRESS

26 GETTING ENOUGH REST

As your baby grows larger, you will suffer from fatigue. If you are still working, it is especially important to have enough rest. Establish a routine of putting your feet up, or taking a nap, after lunch. During the last weeks you will become tired very easily. Don't fight this tiredness. Relax and rest as much as possible.

- Sit down and put your feet up whenever you feel the need to.
- Do your chores at a slower pace so that you don't become overtired.
- Practice relaxation and breathing techniques (*see pp.54–57*) whenever you feel tired or stressed.

REST IS IMPORTANT
Take a regular rest during the day.

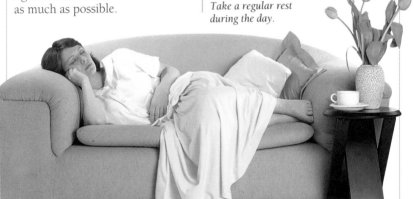

27 EATING SENSIBLY

Eating well while still at work means planning ahead. Buy whole-wheat rolls for lunch. Store mineral water, unsweetened fruit juice, yogurt, cheese, tomatoes, and milk in the office refrigerator. Keep a supply of nuts, seeds, and dried fruit in your drawer for snacks. If there is no refrigerator, bring in a thermos of milk or fruit juice plus homemade sandwiches.

28 KEEPING TEETH & GUMS HEALTHY

You may experience problems with your gums during pregnancy, but a balanced diet, including a good supply of calcium, should help. Visit your dentist at least once during pregnancy to have your teeth professionally cleaned, but be sure to mention you are pregnant since you will be advised to avoid X-rays and anesthetics.

29 AVOIDING STRESS: YOGA

Yoga exercises lessen the effects of such problems as stress and backache, and promote good health in both the mother and the unborn child. Most women who practice yoga find that it can make labor shorter and easier. The postures also help your body adapt to the many changes affecting it, and most can be adapted as your abdomen becomes larger. Pregnancy is also a very good time for meditation. Do these exercises very gently from the beginning of pregnancy, and stop if you feel any pain or discomfort.

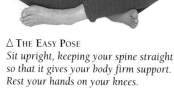

△ THE EASY POSE
Sit upright, keeping your spine straight so that it gives your body firm support. Rest your hands on your knees.

Keep your head back until last. Do not hunch shoulders

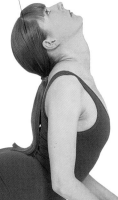

△ FORWARD BEND
Stretch up, lean forward from the hips, and try to touch your toes, or clasp shins or knees. Keep spine and legs straight. Lower your head, but don't force it. Hold for 30 seconds and stretch up. Repeat twice.

STRETCHING YOUR BACK ▷
Lie on your front, feet together, elbows tucked in, forehead on the ground. Slowly roll back and up, keeping the abdomen on the ground, with back arched and chest out. Hold for 10 seconds, then slowly roll down. Repeat 3 times.

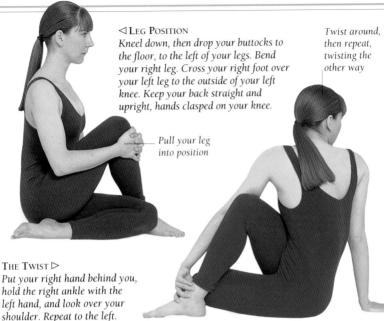

◁ LEG POSITION
Kneel down, then drop your buttocks to the floor, to the left of your legs. Bend your right leg. Cross your right foot over your left leg to the outside of your left knee. Keep your back straight and upright, hands clasped on your knee.

Pull your leg into position

Twist around, then repeat, twisting the other way

THE TWIST ▷
Put your right hand behind you, hold the right ankle with the left hand, and look over your shoulder. Repeat to the left.

FINAL RELAXATION ▽
Lie on your back and close your eyes. Roll your head from side to side, then return to center. Breathe slowly and gently. Stretch out arms and hands, palms upward. Relax jaw and face. Stay for 10 minutes.

SPINAL TWISTING
After bending forward and back, your spine needs a lateral twist to retain its mobility. Try twisting as above from a sitting position first, before attempting the twist from the kneeling position.

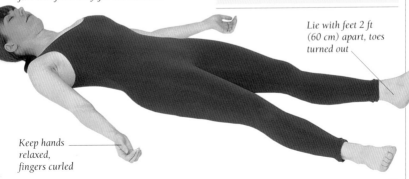

Lie with feet 2 ft (60 cm) apart, toes turned out

Keep hands relaxed, fingers curled

27

AVOIDING INFECTIONS

30 GENERAL ADVICE

There are a number of food-borne and other infections that you should avoid during pregnancy. Probably the best known – and the most common – of these infections is rubella (German measles). Most of the other infectious diseases described in this chapter, although serious, are extremely rare, and if you follow the advice given, the risk of contracting them is slight. Consult your doctor or midwife if you think you are at risk or have any concerns.

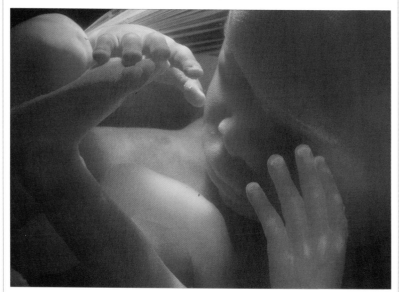

AVOID INFECTIONS THAT MIGHT DAMAGE THE UNBORN BABY

31 RUBELLA

If you catch rubella, or German measles, in pregnancy, especially in the first three months, it can cause serious defects in the fetus, including heart disease, deafness, and blindness. Before you conceive, ask your doctor for a blood test to make sure you are immune to the disease. If you are not, you should be vaccinated. After vaccination, wait for three months before trying to conceive. Tell your doctor at once if you are exposed to rubella.

32 HIV

Women who are already infected with HIV when they become pregnant have a high risk of transmitting the virus to their unborn baby. Infected babies will eventually develop AIDS, and you will therefore be given the option of a termination.

33 TOXOPLASMOSIS

Toxoplasmosis is caused by an organism found in raw meat, and cat and dog feces. It can affect pregnant women, and when the infection is passed to the unborn baby it can cause serious problems, including birth defects.

34 CAT LITTER

Cat litter boxes must be kept clean, but ask someone else to do it if possible. Always wear rubber gloves when changing the litter. Wash the gloves with disinfectant afterward and wash your hands.

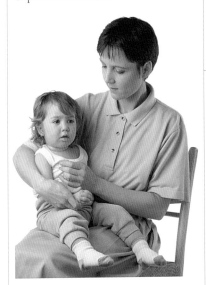

TAKE CARE
If you come into contact with rubella while pregnant, consult your doctor at once to check that you are still immune.

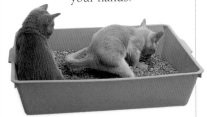

AVOID HANDLING CAT LITTER

35 IN THE GARDEN

Always wash your hands after handling your cats and kittens, no matter how clean they may seem, and avoid contact with other people's cats and kittens. Make sure you always wear gloves when gardening to protect your hands from contamination. Even if you yourself do not keep a cat as a pet, the garden soil may still have been fouled by cats. Always wash

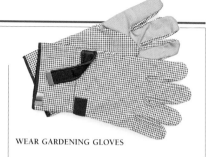

WEAR GARDENING GLOVES

your hands after gardening, even if you have worn gardening gloves, and avoid handling your garden tools without gloves.

36 GOAT'S MILK

Occasionally, goat's milk is found to carry the toxoplasmosis infection (see p.29). If you enjoy drinking goat's milk, it will be safe to continue to do so while you are pregnant, provided that you buy milk that is labeled as guaranteed pasteurized, sterilized, or UHT (ultra-heat-treated). Never drink untreated milk of any kind.

37 VEGETABLES & SALADS

Fresh vegetables, lettuces, and other salad crops should always be washed carefully, even if bought prepared and packaged in a supermarket. If you use homegrown lettuces, cucumbers, tomatoes, and vegetables, or if you buy freshly picked produce from a nursery or farm stand, be particularly careful to wash off any soil or dirt that might carry the infection if it has been fouled by cats. Do not assume that you are safe from infection because you do not have pets; your garden may well be visited by neighborhood pets without your knowledge.

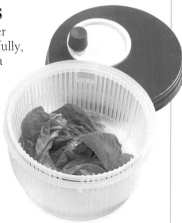

WASH SALADS THOROUGHLY

38 MEAT

Most people contract toxoplasmosis through eating undercooked beef, pork, or poultry. Make sure that meat and poultry is thoroughly defrosted before cooking, then cook to an internal temperature of 140°F/ 54°C, or until the juices run clear when tested with a skewer. Wash hands thoroughly before and after handling raw meat or poultry.

WASH HANDS

39 SICK LAMBS

Sheep may miscarry or give birth to sick lambs following infection with toxoplasmosis. Pregnant women on farms should not help with lambing, milk ewes that have recently given birth, touch the afterbirth, or come into contact with newborn lambs.

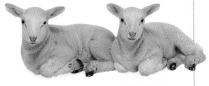

AVOID HANDLING NEWBORN LAMBS

40 BOTULISM

This is a rare but severe form of food poisoning. Improperly canned or preserved food, refrozen packaged food, or spoiled meat, fish, or poultry are usually the culprits. Botulism can cause serious damage to the nervous system.

41 LISTERIOSIS

This illness resembles flu, but even the mild form can cause miscarriage, stillbirth, or severe illness in a newborn baby. It is caused by a bacteria found in some foods (see below and p.32) which you should avoid while pregnant.

42 CHEESE

Some cheeses contain high levels of listeria (see above) and should therefore be avoided if you are pregnant. These are ripened soft cheeses such as Camembert and Brie, and the blue-veined varieties. However, you can still enjoy hard cheeses such as Cheddar, Swiss, and Parmesan, as well as cottage cheese, processed cheese, and cheese spreads.

AVOID SOFT CHEESES

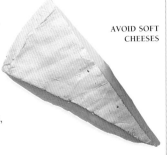

43 PATE

Pâtés are one of the foods that have been found to contain high levels of the listeria bacteria. People who are particularly vulnerable to the infection include the elderly, babies, and pregnant women. Therefore, it is sensible to avoid eating pâtés once you know you are pregnant.

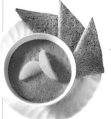

AVOID PATES

44 LEFTOVER FOODS

The listeria bacteria has been found in leftover foods and ready-to-eat poultry. To be on the safe side, either avoid these foods or reheat thoroughly until piping hot, and do not eat them cold.

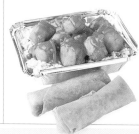

REHEAT UNTIL PIPING HOT

45 SALMONELLA

Salmonella is one of the most common causes of food poisoning. The symptoms include sickness and diarrhea. It is particularly associated with eggs and poultry (see below and right), so take precautions when you are preparing these foods.

46 EGGS

No one should eat raw eggs, or foods containing raw eggs, because of the risk of salmonella, and this advice particularly applies to pregnant women and young children. Choose free-range eggs whenever possible, and cook until both the white and yolk are solid. Discard cracked eggs, and never allow raw egg to come into contact with other food. For recipes containing raw eggs, use liquid or dry pasteurized egg.

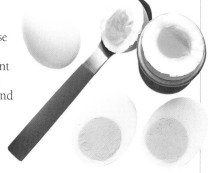

COOK EGGS THOROUGHLY

47 CHICKEN

Poultry can be infected with salmonella bacteria. Heat kills the bacteria, so always cook poultry thoroughly. Defrost birds completely before cooking. Take care not to contaminate other food through contact with raw poultry.

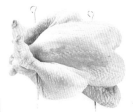

COOK
CHICKEN
THOROUGHLY

48 RAW MEAT

Raw meat can also become infected with salmonella. Like chicken, raw meat should always be handled with care, to avoid contaminating other food. Make sure meat is cooked thoroughly, and do not eat rare beef.

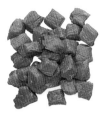

WASH HANDS
AFTER HANDLING
RAW MEAT

49 MILKBORNE INFECTIONS

Milk that has not been heat-treated – that is, it is not pasteurized, sterilized, or UHT – may have been infected with harmful organisms. Unpasteurized milk is sometimes sold in health-food stores or at farms and should be avoided.

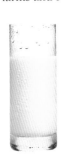

Pasteurized milk still has a high nutritional value and eliminates the risk of infection. As well as milk, you should avoid all dairy products that are unpasteurized.

DRINK PASTEURIZED MILK

50 SAFE FOOD STORAGE

Never take any unnecessary risks when handling and storing food since bacteria can multiply rapidly. Keep food covered, and store cooked and uncooked foods away from each other.

- Store raw poultry on the bottom shelf of the refrigerator and do not allow juices to drip on other foods.
- Defrost poultry in the refrigerator overnight. Make sure the bird is completely defrosted before cooking, or the inside may still be chilled and will not cook through.
- Store raw meat on the bottom shelf of the refrigerator and do not allow it to come into contact with other food.

51 SAFE FOOD PREPARATION

Keep all kitchen work surfaces clean. Always wash your hands before and after preparing food, especially after handling raw meat or poultry. Use two cutting boards, keeping one separate for preparing meat and poultry. Always wash the cutting board and knives after handling raw meat. Try to keep pets out of the kitchen and far away from work surfaces, however well-behaved they are; they may inadvertently spread infection. Prepare pet food apart from other food. Keep special feeding dishes for pets, and wash pet dishes and bowls separately from the rest of your dishes.

CLEAN TOOLS
Always wash knives carefully between jobs, and wash your hands before and after preparing food.

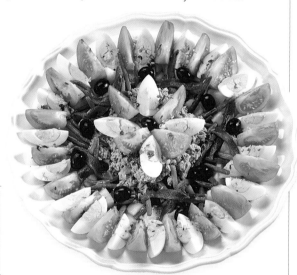

CUTTING BOARDS
Keep a separate cutting board just for preparing raw meat and poultry.

52 COOKING & REHEATING FOOD

Reheat food only once after cooking, and heat thoroughly until it is piping hot all the way through. Always throw away any leftover reheated food. Make sure that frozen food is thoroughly defrosted before cooking, especially poultry, and that it is cooked all the way through. Never refreeze food once it has been defrosted. When using a microwave, observe the standing times recommended in the recipe.

HARMFUL SUBSTANCES

53 GENERAL ADVICE

Once you are pregnant, the effect of anything you eat, drink, smoke, or inhale is likely to cross from your blood into your baby's blood via the placenta. Many substances can harm the baby, especially during the first three months of pregnancy, when the limbs, brain, and internal organs are being formed. For safety's sake, don't take any medicines unless they have been prescribed by a doctor who knows you are pregnant (see p.11). Smoking, alcohol, and "recreational" drugs should likewise be avoided.

IN THE WOMB
The baby in the uterus depends completely on you for the food and oxygen necessary for growth.

The placenta forms a support system that supplies the nutrients to the baby

The umbilical cord links the placenta to the baby. It carries nutrients and blood to the fetus, and transfers away waste products

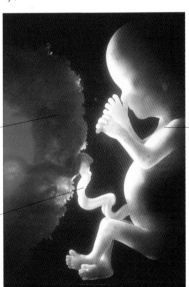

The baby lies curled in the uterus, cushioned by the warm amniotic fluid that protects against infections and sudden bumps

SUPPORT SYSTEM
Almost all the substances that enter your body, good or bad, are filtered through to the baby via the placenta.

54 X-RAYS

X-rays should be avoided during pregnancy because they represent a risk to the developing fetus. Always mention that you are pregnant when you visit the dentist, or if a doctor or other medical professional suggests an X-ray for any reason. If your occupation involves using X-ray machines, or brings you into close proximity with them, ask to be transferred to another department for the duration of your pregnancy.

55 MEDICINES

Once you are pregnant, consult your doctor before taking any drug, prescription, or over-the-counter remedy. Never consult a doctor or dentist about anything without saying you are pregnant. It is best to avoid taking anything while pregnant unless your doctor decides that the benefit to you outweighs the risk to the fetus. The long-term effect of many drugs is unknown, while others are known to be hazardous (*see p. 11*).

56 ALCOHOL & ALTERNATIVES

Any alcohol that you drink during pregnancy is passed through the placenta into the baby's bloodstream. No one knows what the safe limit is, so it is best to avoid alcohol altogether, and make your own fresh fruit "cocktails," milkshakes, and sparkling mineral water drinks. Even beers, lagers, and wines that claim to be alcohol-free, or low in alcohol, are not necessarily free from harmful additives and chemicals, which may have adverse effects on your baby's health.

ALTERNATIVES
Try fresh orange juice diluted with sparkling mineral water for a simple, refreshing drink. Make high-protein milkshakes with banana or other fruits. Mix your own cocktail of fresh fruit juices, and garnish with orange slices.

FRUIT COCKTAIL

SPARKLING ORANGE

MILKSHAKE

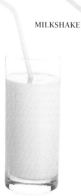
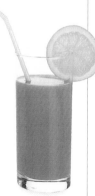

57 CAFFEINE

Coffee, tea, colas, and hot chocolate all contain caffeine, which is believed to have harmful effects. Reduce your intake to no more than two cups of any drink containing caffeine, and if possible cut it out altogether. Drink mineral water instead, or quench your thirst with fruit juices. Prepackaged herbal teas can be a good substitute, but check with a pharmacist or herbalist to see which ones are recommended.

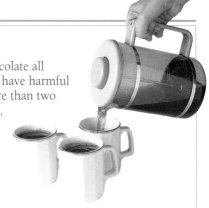

AVOID CAFFEINE

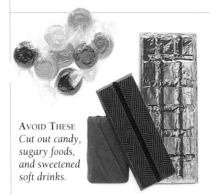

AVOID THESE
Cut out candy, sugary foods, and sweetened soft drinks.

58 EMPTY CALORIES

Cut down on sugary foods, such as cakes, fruit pies, cookies, pastries, jam, soda and other sweetened drinks, canned fruit in syrup, candy and chocolate, and ice creams. These are all low in nutrients, contain only sugar or sugar substitutes, and will make you gain excess weight that you may have trouble shedding later.

59 CIGARETTES

As explained in Thinking about Pregnancy (*see p.10*), smoking can damage the fetus and result in miscarriages. If you are still smoking when you become pregnant, you must try very hard to cut down, and preferably give up cigarettes completely. Even passive smoking can damage you and your baby's health .

60 RECREATIONAL DRUGS

All recreational drugs should be avoided since they are going to affect the baby. Smoking marijuana can affect the baby just as tobacco smoking does. Smoking cocaine or crack affects the baby's oxygen supply, and babies born to women who are addicted to heroin may themselves be addicted at birth.

STAYING IN SHAPE

61 STAYING FIT & RELAXED

Pregnancy and labor will make great demands on your body, so the more you prepare yourself physically, the better you will feel. You will also find it easier to regain your figure after the birth if you keep fit.

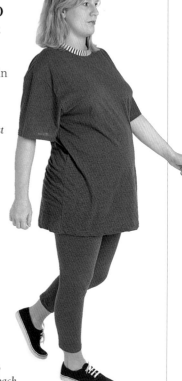

WALKING ▷
This is one of the best ways to get in shape and stay in shape.

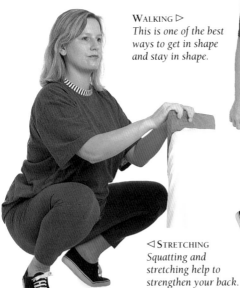

◁ STRETCHING
Squatting and stretching help to strengthen your back.

62 EXERCISING SAFELY

If you have always enjoyed sports, you can usually continue in pregnancy, but remember that it is not the time for a fitness blitz; just continue what your body is used to. Don't exercise to the point where you get breathless or very tired. Swimming is excellent.

63 IMPORTANCE OF GOOD POSTURE

During pregnancy you should be conscious of standing straight and avoiding strain on your back. The baby's weight pulls you forward, which results in a tendency to lean backward to compensate. This strains the muscles of the lower back and pelvis, especially near the end of your term. Be aware of your body whatever you are doing, and avoid heavy lifting. Wear low heels; high heels throw your weight even farther forward.

Drop your shoulders and keep them back

Lift your chest and ribs

Hold your back straight

Tighten your stomach

Tuck in your bottom

GOOD POSTURE ▷
Lengthen and straighten your back, so that the weight of the baby is centered and supported by your thighs, buttocks, and stomach muscles. This will prevent backache.

Bend your knees slightly

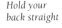

◁ BAD POSTURE
As the baby grows, its weight throws you off-balance, so you may overarch your back and thrust your abdomen forward.

Stand with your feet a little way apart

64 PROTECTING YOUR BACK

During pregnancy, you are much more likely to suffer from backache. Hormones make the muscles of the lower back stretch and soften, and so they are much more easily strained if you bend over, get up too suddenly, or lift something in the wrong way.

Avoid bending over

65 LOW LEVEL WORKING

Do as much as you can at floor level. Instead of bending over, kneel down to weed the garden. Kneel down to do the housework, too, whenever possible, especially when making beds. If you have small children to care for, kneel down to dress or feed them. At work too, kneel down to reach low file drawers, or to pick up piles of papers or books.

KNEELING DOWN
Whenever possible, kneel down rather than bend over, which puts a strain on your back.

66 LIFTING & CARRYING

When lifting something heavy, bend your knees and crouch down. Keep your back as straight as possible and bring the weight close in to your body. Lift slowly and smoothly, using the strength of your leg and thigh muscles to do the work. Try not to lift heavy objects to or from a high shelf, as you may lose your balance. To carry heavy bags, divide the weight equally between both hands.

CORRECT POSITION
The right way to lift something heavy is to get down to it. Bend your knees and keep your back straight.

Keep your back straight when lifting

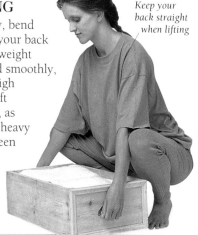

67 GETTING UP

When you have been lying down on the floor, exercising or doing relaxation techniques, get up in easy stages. Always turn onto your side when you have been lying down. Then move into a kneeling position. Use the strength of your thighs to push yourself up.

1 ◁ From lying down flat on the floor, first turn onto your side, leaning on one elbow, and crossing the upper leg over the lower one.

Turn onto your side

Cross your upper leg over the lower

2 ▷ Support yourself with your hands as you move into a kneeling position. Sit upright with your back straight.

3 ▷ Use the strength of your thighs to push yourself up, keeping your back straight.

41

68 BACK EXERCISES

These exercises relieve the strain caused by your extra weight and strengthen important muscles. They also increase circulation and can help relieve tension. Labor may be easier and more comfortable if you have good muscle tone, and you will find it easier to return to your prepregnancy weight. Try to adopt a regular exercise routine. Begin gently and gradually build up to what feels right. Several short spells of exercise are better than one long session. Stop if you suffer pain, cramping, or shortness of breath.

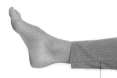

Keep the other leg flat on the floor

1 ▽ Lie flat on your back with arms by your sides, palms down. Press your feet into the floor. Breathe in and lift your pelvis and spine off the floor; then slowly breathe out as you lower your back.

Raise yourself on supported arms

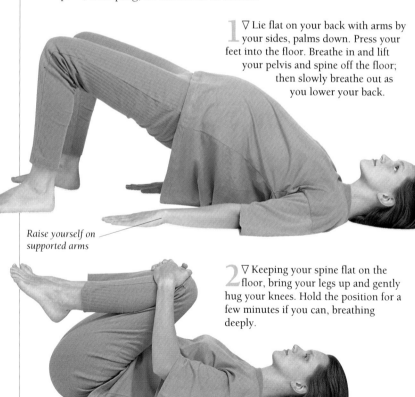

2 ▽ Keeping your spine flat on the floor, bring your legs up and gently hug your knees. Hold the position for a few minutes if you can, breathing deeply.

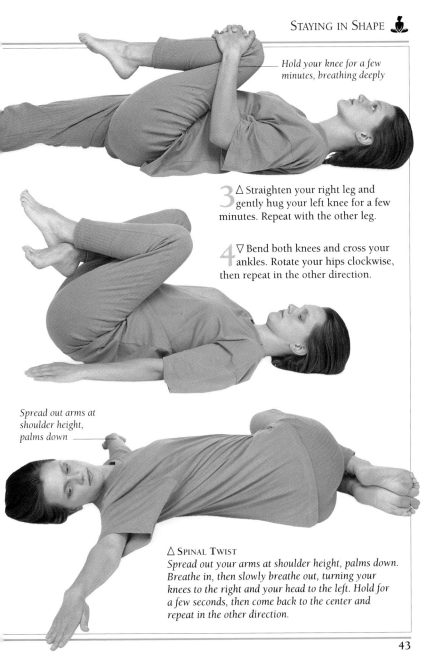

Hold your knee for a few minutes, breathing deeply

3 △ Straighten your right leg and gently hug your left knee for a few minutes. Repeat with the other leg.

4 ▽ Bend both knees and cross your ankles. Rotate your hips clockwise, then repeat in the other direction.

Spread out arms at shoulder height, palms down

△ SPINAL TWIST
Spread out your arms at shoulder height, palms down. Breathe in, then slowly breathe out, turning your knees to the right and your head to the left. Hold for a few seconds, then come back to the center and repeat in the other direction.

69 STRETCHING

These stretching exercises are invaluable as a way of relieving tension or fatigue. They are easy to do and fit into your normal daily routine. The gentle movements are designed to warm up your muscles and joints, thus stimulating your circulation and improving the supply of oxygen both for you and your baby. Always wear comfortable clothes and make sure that your back is straight before you begin. Stop if you feel pain or discomfort.

△ HEAD & NECK
Gently tilt your head to one side and down, feeling the stretch on the side of your neck. Bring your head up and tilt over to the other side. Repeat 5 times.

◁ WAIST
Sit crosslegged and turn to the right. Look back and place your right hand behind you. Place your left hand on your right knee to twist farther. Repeat, turning to the left.

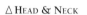

Place your hand on your knee to help twist farther

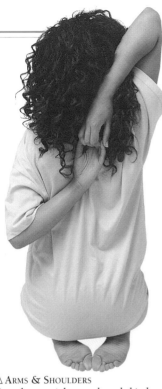

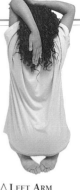

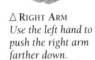

△ **Right Arm**
Use the left hand to push the right arm farther down.

△ **Left Arm**
Repeat the exercise with the left arm stretched down.

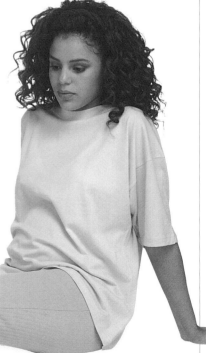

△ **Arms & Shoulders**
Stretch your right arm down behind your back. Put your left hand on your elbow and push it farther down, then put your left arm behind your back and grasp your right hand. Hold for 20 seconds, then relax.

▽ **Legs & Feet**
Sit with your legs stretched out and your hands on the floor to help support your weight. Bend one knee slowly, then straighten. Repeat with the other knee.

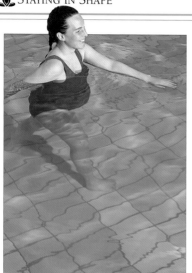

70 SWIMMING

Swimming is highly beneficial when you are pregnant, both as an aid to relaxation and as a pleasant way of exercising safely. In late pregnancy the support that the water gives you will be particularly enjoyable. Apart from floating, all the exercises shown here and on pp.48–49 can be carried out even if you cannot swim. Be careful not to arch your back when swimming. If you have back trouble, avoid the breaststroke and do sidestroke or backstroke.

Swing your arm high

△ **WARM-UP**
Begin by striding across the pool at the shallow end, lifting each leg high and stretching it out in front of you as you walk.

SWING YOUR ARMS ▷
Swing your arms as you stride, as if you were marching, stretching the opposite arm high in the air with each step.

STRIDING OUT
Striding is surprisingly difficult against the resistance of the water. Walk backward and forward across the pool a few times, breathing deeply and slowly, but do not tire yourself out.

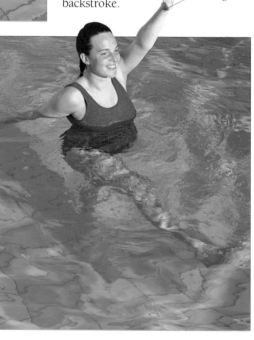

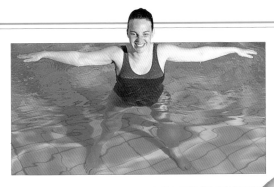

◁ STRETCHING
This is an ideal exercise for keeping your joints supple and relaxed. Start by standing at the shallow end with your back against the rail. Stand with your feet well apart and your arms outstretched.

BENDING ▷
Now stretch your right arm over your head, bend it toward the left one and try to touch it. Sway over to the other side and repeat.

FLOATING ▽
Take a deep breath and push your pelvis up so you are lying flat on the water, arms outstretched.

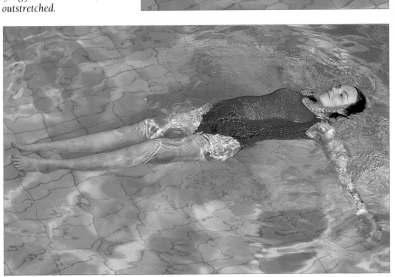

71 SIDE OF THE POOL EXERCISES

These exercises can be performed at the shallow end of the pool and are safe even for a nonswimmer. However, you should have someone with you just in case you have problems or have trouble getting out of the pool. Start by doing the warm-up striding exercise (see p.46) to stimulate your circulation. Do each exercise four or five times, but stop if you are getting tired or out of breath. If you are a good swimmer, floating (see p.47) is a good way of relaxing between each different exercise. You may find it helpful to place a float between your legs or under your pelvis.

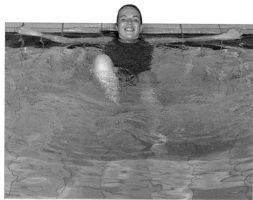

◁ CYCLING
Stand with your back to the wall and hold on with arms outstretched. Raise your legs until you are floating on your back, then move your legs as if cycling in the water. Do this exercise slowly for about two minutes, bending and stretching your legs as vigorously as possible in the water.

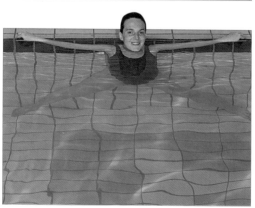

◁ STRETCHING SIDEWAYS
Again stand with your back to the wall and hold on to it with your arms outstretched. Keeping your back pressed against the side, slide your legs apart as far as possible, so that your body slides down into the water. You will feel the pull on your thighs. Bring your legs together again and repeat the movement four or five times.

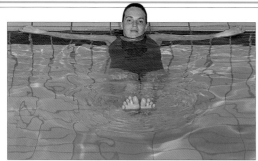

◁ STRETCH & SQUAT
Stand against the wall and hold on to it with your arms outstretched as before. Stretch your legs straight out directly in front of you until they are floating in the water, then bend your knees right up to your body in a squatting position.

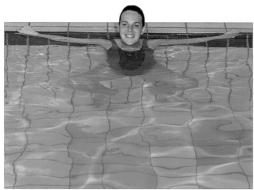

◁ FROG MOVEMENT
Take up the squatting position (above) then move your legs out to the sides as far as possible, keeping your knees bent, until you feel the stretch on your inner thighs. Bring your legs together again, stretch them out in front, then again take up the squatting position and repeat the exercise three or four times.

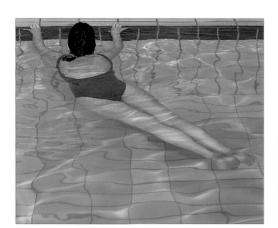

◁ SWINGING SIDEWAYS
Face the edge and hold on to the rail, just slightly out of your depth. Gently swing your legs from side to side, bending from the waist. Repeat ten times as smoothly as possible.

SWIM ON YOUR BACK
If you prefer swimming, try swimming on your back with breaststroke leg movements, arms copying leg movements.

49

PREPARING FOR LABOR

72 PELVIC FLOOR

This is a hammock of muscles that supports the bowel, bladder, and uterus. In pregnancy, the muscles turn soft and stretchy and this, with the weight of the baby, weakens them. You may leak urine when you cough or sneeze.

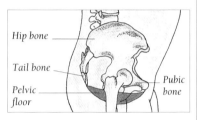

Hip bone

Tail bone

Pelvic floor

Pubic bone

PELVIC FLOOR

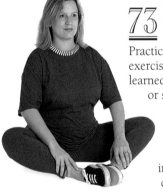

SIT, LIE, OR STAND

73 PELVIC FLOOR EXERCISE

Practice pelvic floor exercises (also called Kegel exercises) several times a day. Once you have learned it, you can do it anywhere, lying, sitting, or standing. Lie or sit on the floor, knees bent and feet flat or in the tailor position (*see p.52*). Now tighten the muscles, squeezing. Imagine you are trying to pull something into your vagina. Draw it in slightly, then pause, then pull until you can go no farther. Hold for a moment, then let go gradually. Repeat ten times.

74 WHEN TO DO THE EXERCISE

You can perform the pelvic floor exercise while waiting for a bus or train, sitting at a desk, while ironing or cooking, watching TV, while having intercourse, or after you have emptied your bladder.

75 PELVIC TILT

This exercise helps you move your pelvis with ease, which is a good preparation for labor. It is especially helpful if you suffer from backaches, and when you are in the all-fours position your partner can rub the base of your back to soothe your pain. You can carry out the tilt in any position, sitting, standing, or kneeling. Try to keep your shoulders still.

Hold your back flat to start with

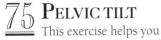

1 ◁ Kneel on the floor on your hands and knees. Make sure that your back is flat – it helps to do this in front of a mirror at first to check that your position is correct.

2 ▷ Pull in your stomach muscles, tighten your buttocks, and gently tilt the pelvis forward, breathing out as you do so. Your back should arch up. Hold this position for a few seconds, then breathe in and let go. Repeat several times, so that your pelvis is rocking.

Keep your arms straight and hands flat on the floor

76 TAILOR SITTING

This strengthens your back and makes your thighs and pelvis more flexible, helpful if you give birth in a squatting position, which some women find easier. It also improves blood flow in the lower part of your body and makes your joints more supple. The position is easier than it looks, as your body is more supple during pregnancy.

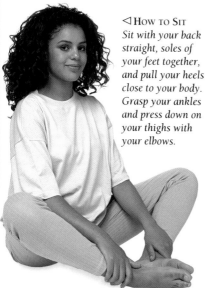

◁ HOW TO SIT
Sit with your back straight, soles of your feet together, and pull your heels close to your body. Grasp your ankles and press down on your thighs with your elbows.

◁ CORRECT
Put your feet together at the distance from your body where it feels comfortable, and gradually pull them in closer.

◁ INCORRECT
It is important to sit with a straight back while performing this exercise. Relax your shoulders and neck.

77 SITTING WITH CUSHIONS

If you find tailor sitting difficult at first, put a cushion under each thigh, or sit against a wall for support if you find it easier. Remember to keep your back straight.

USE CUSHIONS FOR SUPPORT

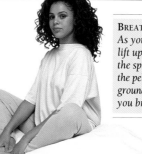

BREATHING
As you breathe in, lift up and stretch the spine, keeping the pelvis on the ground. Relax as you breathe out.

78 WHEN TO SQUAT

Squatting increases the flexibility of the pelvic joints and strengthens the back and thigh muscles. It can protect your back if you squat instead of bending.

- Squat to relieve back pain.
- Try it when you feel breathless.
- Squat rather than bend over.
- Squat if lifting something heavy.
- Squat if no chair is available.

79 SQUATTING WITH A CHAIR

Squatting exercises are very useful during pregnancy. The exercise fully stretches the pelvis and helps to relax the tissues. Some women also find it easier to give birth in a squatting position. You may find it difficult to do a full squat at first (see p.54), so try holding on to a firm support, such as a chair or a windowsill, and place a rolled-up rug or blanket under your heels. Get up slowly from the squatting position, or you may make yourself dizzy.

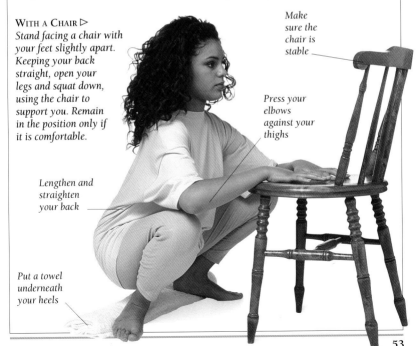

WITH A CHAIR ▷
Stand facing a chair with your feet slightly apart. Keeping your back straight, open your legs and squat down, using the chair to support you. Remain in the position only if it is comfortable.

Make sure the chair is stable

Press your elbows against your thighs

Lengthen and straighten your back

Put a towel underneath your heels

53

80 SQUATTING UNSUPPORTED

After some practice at squatting holding onto a support (*see p.53*), you can try a full squat without support. Keeping your back straight, open out your legs and squat down, turning your feet out slightly. Try to keep your heels flat on the ground and stretch your inner thighs by pressing outward with your elbows. Stay in this position for as long as it feels comfortable.

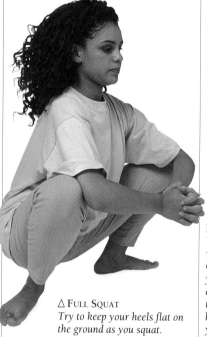

△ FULL SQUAT
Try to keep your heels flat on the ground as you squat.

81 THE LATE STAGES OF PREGNANCY

As you become larger in the last few weeks, sitting or lying in your usual positions will become very uncomfortable. If you lie flat on your back, the weight of the baby presses down on the major blood vessels and nerves of the spine, causing numbness and tingling. Prop yourself up with cushions or pillows to support your body, then try the tense and relax technique, which is a good preparation for labor. This involves first tensing and then relaxing different parts of your body in sequence. Start with the right hand, arm, and shoulder, then the left, then the buttocks, thighs, calves, and feet. Finally, relax your head, neck, and face. Do this twice a day for 15 minutes.

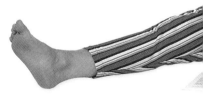

RESTING ON YOUR BACK ▷
Try the tense and relax technique (above) while lying propped up with cushions. Close your eyes and breathe slowly. When your mind is relaxed and your breathing deep and regular, start the exercise, beginning with your right hand.

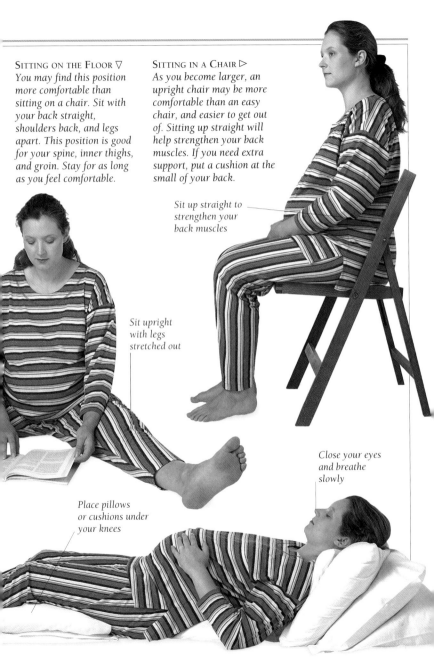

SITTING ON THE FLOOR ▽
You may find this position more comfortable than sitting on a chair. Sit with your back straight, shoulders back, and legs apart. This position is good for your spine, inner thighs, and groin. Stay for as long as you feel comfortable.

SITTING IN A CHAIR ▷
As you become larger, an upright chair may be more comfortable than an easy chair, and easier to get out of. Sitting up straight will help strengthen your back muscles. If you need extra support, put a cushion at the small of your back.

Sit up straight to strengthen your back muscles

Sit upright with legs stretched out

Close your eyes and breathe slowly

Place pillows or cushions under your knees

82 RELAXATION & BREATHING EXERCISES

These exercises are invaluable during labor, when knowing how to breathe properly and relax the muscles will help you cope with contractions and save vital energy. Practice them regularly so that they become a natural response during labor. Relaxation will help you unwind at any time you feel tense or anxious. Start by tensing and relaxing each muscle in turn (*see p.54*). After eight to ten minutes, let your body go limp and heavy, as though you are sinking into the floor.

Now practice your breathing – breathe in and out of your mouth, taking very light, shallow breaths – this light breathing is helpful at the height of a contraction. Now breathe in deeply, right to the bottom of your lungs, and breathe out slowly and gently. This has a calming effect after contractions.

WARNING
Never lie flat on your back in the late stages of pregnancy; this restricts the flow of oxygen to the baby, and you may feel faint. In any case, you will probably find it extremely uncomfortable without some support.

LYING ON YOUR SIDE ▽
During late pregnancy you may find it more comfortable lying on your side, with one leg bent and supported by cushions. Do not place too many pillows under your head, as this is bad for your spine

Pull in your
stomach muscles,
then relax

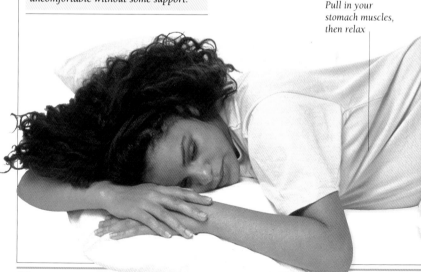

83 RELAXING YOUR MIND

While relaxing your body, try to calm and empty your mind. Breathe slowly and evenly, sighing each breath out gently. Do not breathe too hard. Try repeating a word or sound to yourself, or concentrate on some pleasant or peaceful image. Ignore any stressful thoughts or anxieties that come into your mind and try to concentrate solely on your breathing.

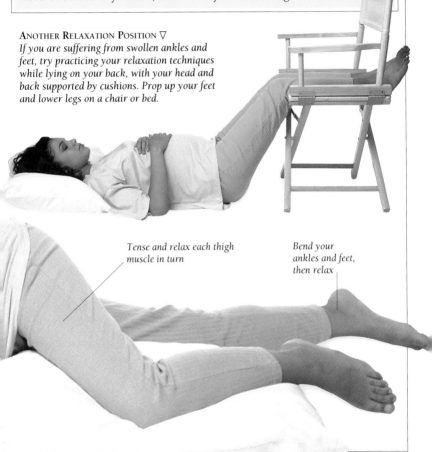

ANOTHER RELAXATION POSITION ▽
If you are suffering from swollen ankles and feet, try practicing your relaxation techniques while lying on your back, with your head and back supported by cushions. Prop up your feet and lower legs on a chair or bed.

Tense and relax each thigh muscle in turn

Bend your ankles and feet, then relax

COMMON COMPLAINTS

84 BREATHLESSNESS

During the later stages of pregnancy, the growing baby puts pressure on the diaphragm and prevents you from breathing freely. The problem is often relieved about a month before the birth, when the baby's head engages. Breathlessness can also be caused by anemia. The solution is to rest as much as possible. Try crouching if you feel breathless when there is no chair nearby.

CROUCHING
If you suddenly feel out of breath halfway up the stairs, hold onto the bannister and crouch until the feeling has passed.

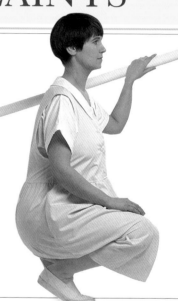

85 SKIN & NAILS

The skin usually improves during pregnancy, but it may become very dry and scaly, or oily. Always cleanse your skin thoroughly, but avoid using soap. If skin is dry, use a moisturizer and add bath oils to your bath. Don't worry if your skin color darkens, especially freckles and moles, or if you develop dark patches. This disappears after the birth. Wear gloves if your nails split and break easily.

SKIN PIGMENTATION MAY CHANGE

86 CRAMPS

Leg cramps often strike at night, giving painful contractions of the muscles in the calves and feet. The best remedy to improve your circulation is to massage the affected leg or foot, then walk around once the pain has eased. Cramps can be caused by a calcium deficiency. See your doctor, who may prescribe calcium and vitamin D supplements.

MASSAGE FOR CRAMPS
Pull your foot up toward you and massage the calf vigorously.

87 SWOLLEN ANKLES

Some swelling is normal since the body holds extra water in pregnancy and this is usually no cause for concern. You may have slight swelling in the ankles, especially in hot weather and at the end of the day. The answer is to rest with your feet up as often as possible. You can also try gentle foot exercises to improve circulation. See your doctor or midwife if it gets worse. More marked swelling could be a warning sign of preeclampsia, which causes raised blood pressure.

FOOT EXERCISES
To relieve swollen ankles, gently circle your ankles and feet to improve the circulation.

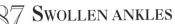

88 VARICOSE VEINS

You are more likely to develop varicose veins if you are overweight, or if they run in your family. Standing for too long can make the problem worse. The veins become painful and swollen, and your legs ache. Rest with your feet up whenever possible, and wear support hose.

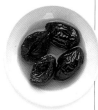

Prop your feet up

VARICOSE VEINS
Rest with your feet raised on a chair with at least two cushions. Tuck another cushion behind your back.

89 CONSTIPATION

This is a very common problem, but diet and exercise will probably remedy it. Do not take laxatives; see your doctor if the problem persists.

△ DRIED FRUIT

△ VEGETABLES

REMEDIES
Eat plenty of high-fiber foods, including vegetables, dried fruit, and whole-grain bread and cereals, and drink plenty of water. Get regular exercise.

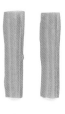

△ CARROTS

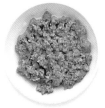

△ WHOLE-GRAIN CEREALS

△ PRUNES

90 HEARTBURN

Heartburn is common because of hormonal changes during pregnancy. The strong burning pain in your chest is very unpleasant and may add to your sleeping problems. To prevent heartburn, avoid large meals and highly spiced or fried food. Try warm milk at night and sleep propped up with extra pillows. Do not take indigestion remedies without consulting your doctor. He or she may prescribe an antacid for stomach acidity, but is unlikely to prescribe sleeping pills.

91 NAUSEA & MORNING SICKNESS

This is often one of the first signs of pregnancy, and it can occur at any time of day. Tiredness can make the problem worse. Nausea usually disappears after the 12th week, but sometimes returns later. Avoid foods and smells that make you feel sick, such as cigarette smoke. Have small, frequent meals during the day. To counteract nausea, try eating a dry cracker, dry toast, or fruit. Ginger cookies or ginger ale can be helpful, as can mineral water.

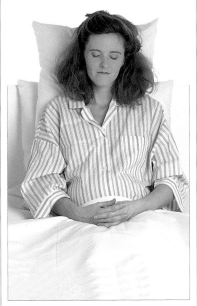

PROP YOURSELF UP WITH PILLOWS

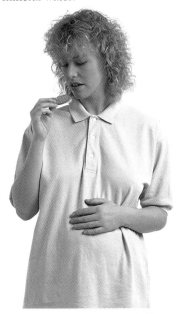

TRY DRY CRACKERS OR TOAST

92 OTHER COMMON COMPLAINTS

You may suffer from a variety of discomforts in pregnancy (the most common ones are discussed on pp.58–61). These complaints, although troublesome at the time, are perfectly normal. Many are caused by hormonal changes or by the extra pressure on your body. A few symptoms may indicate something more serious; always consult your doctor if you suffer severe headache, blurred vision, stomach pains, vaginal bleeding, or frequent vomiting.

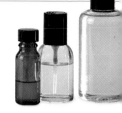

AROMATHERAPY
Massage with oils helps to relax your mind and body.

Complaint	Why it happens	What can be done
Backache	Caused by softening and stretching of the pelvic bones to allow the baby to be born	Improved posture (*see p.39*), massage, and gentle exercises (*see pp.40–43*) will all help
Bleeding gums, especially after brushing your teeth	The gums are softer in pregnancy and may become inflamed, which can lead to gum disease and tooth decay	Floss and brush your teeth thoroughly after eating. See your dentist if you experience severe problems, and do not miss regular check-ups
Diarrhea	Caused by an infection or virus	Increase your water intake to replace lost fluid. Consult your doctor if it persists
Feeling faint	Blood pressure is lower in pregnancy	Sit down and put head between knees. Stand up slowly from a hot bath, or when lying down
Frequent urination	Caused by uterus pressing on the bladder	Try drinking less at night
Hemorrhoids	Baby pressing down on rectum causes swollen rectal veins	Avoid straining and eat plenty of fiber. Your doctor can give ointment to relieve itching

Complaint	Why it happens	What can be done
Insomnia	Size of the bulge makes it difficult to get comfortable in bed	Relaxation exercises (see pp. 40–43). Try sleeping propped up, or with a pillow under one leg.
Painful breasts	Hormonal changes	Wear a good support bra. Do not use soap on nipples
Rash under the breasts or in the groin	Usually in women who are overweight	Wash frequently with nonperfumed soap and apply calamine lotion. Wear loose cotton clothes
Red stretch marks on thighs, stomach, or breasts, fading to silvery streaks	Skin stretched beyond normal elasticity. Being overweight can be a factor	Gain weight gradually. Oils and creams will soothe the skin but will not prevent marks
Sweating after little exertion. Waking up feeling hot and sweaty	Hormonal changes	Wear loose cotton clothes and drink plenty of water
Water retention, causing swelling of the hands, feet and face. Rings may be tight	Standing a lot can cause fluid to gather. Hormonal changes cause retention of sodium	Avoid standing for long periods, and rest with your feet up when possible. Avoid eating salty foods
Yeast infection – white vaginal discharge and severe itching	Hormonal changes	Avoid wearing tight panty hose or pants. Wear cotton rather than man-made fibers. Consult your doctor

TRY NOT TO WORRY
Most complaints are perfectly normal. Staying calm and relaxed will help.

AFTER THE BIRTH

93 POSTPARTUM EXERCISES

With some gentle exercising every day, your figure can return to normal in as little as three months, although your stomach muscles may not be as firm as before. You can begin to strengthen the muscles of your pelvic floor (*see pp.50–51*) and stomach from the first day after birth. Build up slowly at first.

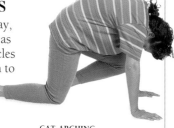

CAT ARCHING

94 STOMACH TONER

Do this from day five after birth. Lie on your back with head and shoulders on two pillows, legs bent and slightly apart. Cross your arms over your stomach. Lift your head and shoulders, breathing out, and press gently on each side of the stomach with your hands. Hold for a few seconds, then breathe in and relax. Repeat three times.

WARNING
If you have had a cesarean, wait 4–6 weeks before doing this exercise.

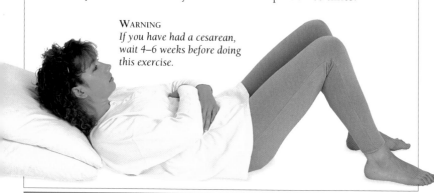

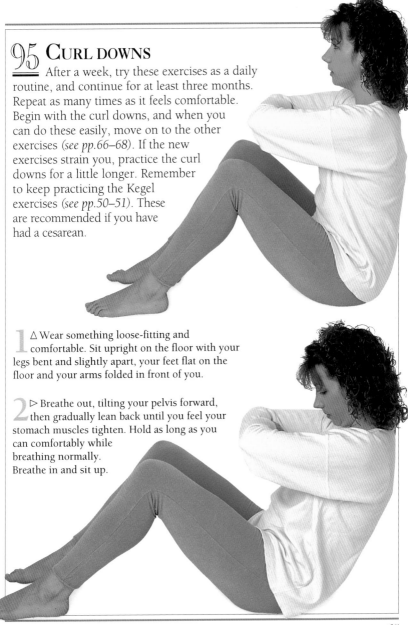

95 CURL DOWNS

After a week, try these exercises as a daily routine, and continue for at least three months. Repeat as many times as it feels comfortable. Begin with the curl downs, and when you can do these easily, move on to the other exercises (see pp.66–68). If the new exercises strain you, practice the curl downs for a little longer. Remember to keep practicing the Kegel exercises (see pp.50–51). These are recommended if you have had a cesarean.

1 △ Wear something loose-fitting and comfortable. Sit upright on the floor with your legs bent and slightly apart, your feet flat on the floor and your arms folded in front of you.

2 ▷ Breathe out, tilting your pelvis forward, then gradually lean back until you feel your stomach muscles tighten. Hold as long as you can comfortably while breathing normally. Breathe in and sit up.

96 CURL UPS

When you can do curl downs easily, try curl ups. Lie flat on your back on the floor, knees bent and feet flat on the floor, slightly apart. Rest your hands on your thighs. Breathe out and lift your head and shoulders, stretching forward to touch your knees with your hands. Breathe in and relax. When this is easy, come up more slowly and hold the position longer. Place your hands on your chest as you lift your head and shoulders, then clasp them behind your head.

TOUCHING YOUR KNEES
Don't worry if you cannot reach your knees at first – you will with practice.

97 SIDE STRETCH

Try this after the curl ups. Lie flat on your back with your arms by your side, and the palms of your hands resting on the outside of your thighs. Lift your head slightly and, bending to the left, slide your left hand down your leg. Lie back and rest for a minute, then repeat on the right side. As this becomes easy, try bending to each side two or three times before you lie back and rest.

STRETCHING TO THE LEFT
Slide your left hand down your leg as far as possible.

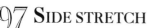

98 LIMBERING UP

Now try cat arching. Kneel on all fours with your back straight. Breathing in, bend one leg up and lower your forehead toward your knee. Hold for a second. Breathing out, stretch, raising your leg behind you and lifting up your head. Hold the pose for a few seconds, then repeat with the other leg.

Stretch your neck and push your chin forward

CAT ARCHING ▷
This is a more strenuous exercise. Your thigh muscles contract and stretch in a steady rhythm as you first bend your knee and then stretch your leg behind you.

Feel your thigh muscles stretch

Keep knees bent and feet flat on the floor

ABDOMINAL TONER ▽
Lie on your back on the floor, knees bent and arms by your sides. Breathe deeply. As you breathe out, raise your head and arms, palms upward. Hold for a few seconds, then relax.

99 BENDING

After a few weeks, get into a regular exercise routine. It's better to do a few exercises twice a day, rather than a long session. You may feel there is no time, but exercising will increase your energy levels and improve your morale. Continue with the exercises on pages 65–66 and start these bending exercises, which will help to recover your waistline. Try the exercises after the bathing and feeding routine – your baby will find it entertaining!

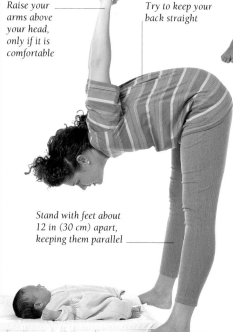

Feel the pull on your side

Gently slide your hand down your leg

Raise your arms above your head, only if it is comfortable

Try to keep your back straight

Stand with feet about 12 in (30 cm) apart, keeping them parallel

△ SIDE BENDS
With feet apart, slowly bend over to the right, raising your left arm over your head and sliding the right hand down your leg. Repeat on other side.

◁ FORWARD BENDS
Clasp your hands behind your back. Bend forward, raising your hands as high as possible.

WARNING
If you have had a cesarean, or stitches following a tear or an episiotomy, consult with your doctor before starting to do any exercises.

100 TESTING PELVIC FLOOR MUSCLES

If you do the Kegel exercises (*see pp.50–51*) as often as possible, your pelvic floor muscles should be strong again three months after the birth. Test them by jumping rope. If any urine leaks, practice the exercises for another month and try again. If leaking is still a problem after four months, consult your doctor.

101 HEALTHY EATING WHILE BREAST-FEEDING

All you need to do to produce enough milk is to eat a balanced diet with plenty of protein and fresh fruit and vegetables, as you were eating while pregnant (*see pp.13–23 for advice on nutrients*). Drink whenever you are thirsty – have a glass of milk or orange juice on hand as you nurse the baby – and rest as much as you can. You need a lot of energy to produce milk, so this is not the time to diet: it will just make you feel exhausted.

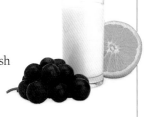

△ BALANCED DIET
Your diet should include fresh fruit and vegetables and plenty of fluids.

DRUGS & MEDICATION
What you eat and drink can be passed on to your baby through your milk, so it is important that you remind your doctor that you are breast-feeding before you take any prescription medicines. You should also avoid stimulants such as caffeine and alcohol. If your baby is restless and does not sleep well, try cutting out all caffeine for a few weeks – the caffeine may be helping to keep or her awake.

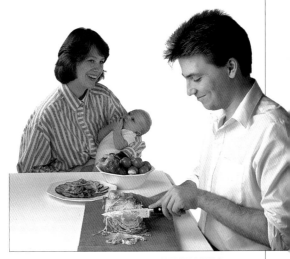

YOUR PARTNER CAN HELP PREPARE MEALS

INDEX

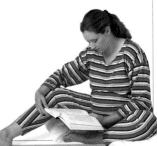

Acknowledgments

Dorling Kindersley would like to thank Hilary Bird for compiling the index, Anne Crane for proofreading, Lesley Malkin for editorial assistance, Murdo Culver for design assistance, and Robert Campbell for page makeup assistance. Special thanks to The Riverside Club, Chiswick, London, and Pippa Blackford for modeling.

Photography
KEY: t *top*; b *bottom*; c *center*; l *left*; r *right*
Ranald Mackechnie: 9, 10, 20, 37, 40-5, 51-7, 62-3, 64t;
Antonia Deutsch: 8, 12-13, 58-9, 60-1, 64b, 65-7;
Andy Crawford: 2, 39, 46-9; Dave King: 14-19, 25, 29, 32tl, 33r, 36, 60b, 69b, 72; David Murray: 21, 22, 31b, 32tl, 33l, 34;
Genesis Film Production/Neil Bromhill: 28, 35; Clive Streeter: 23;
Jane Stockman: 26-7; Gordon Clayton: 32tr; Stephen Oliver: 69t

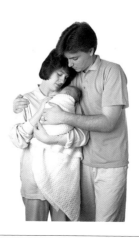